Master Your Muscles

Transform Your Body With Cutting-edge Strategies

By

KR GOSWAMI

Visit:

https://krgoswami.com/titles.html

Let Us Join Hand and Grow Together:

https://krgoswami.com/join-hands.html

This book is dedicated to:

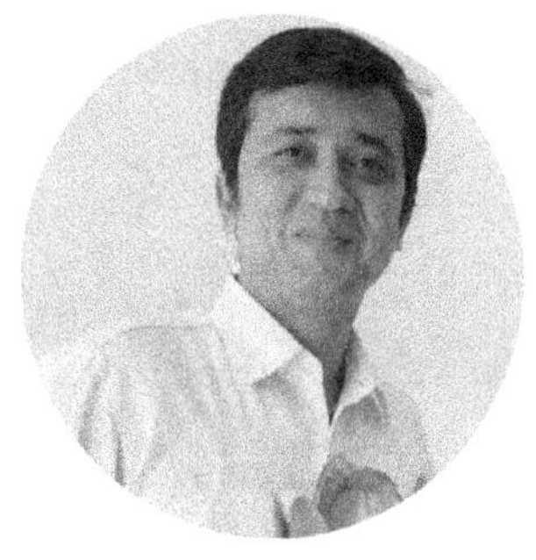

Prashant Goswami, My Nephew

Fitness Enthusiast & Gym Goer

Table of Contents

Introduction

Have you ever wondered if there's an activity that can boost your focus and improve your mood? What if this activity not only has immediate effects but also offers long-term benefits for your brain? Imagine engaging in such an activity that not only protects your brain from ailments like depression, anxiety, and dementia but also provides a powerful solution to enhance your overall well-being. In my book, "Master Your Muscles," I delve into the profound impact of specific physical activities on your entire psychosomatic structure, drawing from my background in psychology and a wealth of experiences.

From my earlier work, I have come to understand that the brain, our most intricate and complex structure, house crucial regions responsible for decision-making, attention, and memory formation. I've always been captivated by the enigmatic hippocampus, a deep region within the temporal lobe, which plays a pivotal role in retaining long-term memories. How is it that seemingly fleeting moments, like the touch of a loved one or the birth of a child, can create memories that last a lifetime?

My research initially focused on uncovering the intricate processes of memory formation, exploring the influence of brief bursts of brain activity between neurons. However, along the way, I experienced a remarkable turning point. Despite my scientific pursuits and scholarly readings, I realized that my personal life was suffering. Loneliness pervaded my military career, as I spent countless solitary hours on helipads and runways, neglecting social connections. But amidst this isolation, my dedication to physical activities and evening gym training provided me with physical and mental well-being, leading me to profound happiness—something I am eager to share with you.

Following my retirement from the Air Force, I embarked on a new journey—a journey that took me back to the gym. I embraced various exercise regimens, ranging from treadmill workouts to yoga sessions. While initially challenging, each sweat-inducing endeavor delivered a substantial boost to my mood and energy, igniting a newfound motivation to persist. As time went on, I grew stronger, shed weight, and then an extraordinary moment occurred. While penning these words, a thought materialized in my mind—one that had never surfaced before: "Today, my ability to focus and sustain attention is unparalleled, and even my long-term memory, the subject of my research, seems to have improved." It struck me that the physical exercise I had incorporated into my life had inadvertently transformed my physical fitness and brain health.

As an inquisitive psychologist, I attribute these remarkable changes to my recent physical activities, prompting me to share my experiences through the pages of this book in a more compelling manner. To my exhilaration, I discovered a growing body of research that substantiated my encounters: exercise enhances mood, energy levels, memory, and attention. The more I delved into this subject, the more I realized the profound power of exercise. This realization led me to make a pivotal decision—shifting my research and writing focus entirely. After years of devoted study, I firmly believe that exercise is the most transformative activity we can engage in to optimize our psychosomatic structure.

In the subsequent chapters of "Master Your Muscles," we will explore the immediate effects of exercise on the brain, from elevating neurotransmitter levels such as dopamine and serotonin to unveiling the long-term benefits that extend far beyond physical fitness. Prepare to embark on a journey of self-discovery as we unravel the science behind exercise's transformative potential.

Chapter 1

Understanding Your Muscles

In our journey toward achieving physical strength and fitness, understanding our muscles is paramount. They are the powerhouses that allow us to move, perform daily tasks, and engage in athletic pursuits. To truly master our muscles and optimize their potential, we must delve into the intricate world of muscle anatomy, physiology, and growth. Let us discuss the foundation, providing a comprehensive overview of the fascinating realm of muscle mastery.

The Anatomy and Physiology of Muscles

Before we can comprehend the complexities of muscle mastery, we need to grasp the fundamental structure and function of our muscles. This will explore the anatomy and physiology of muscles, delving into their composition, organization, and the mechanisms that enable them to contract and generate force. We will examine the different types of muscles, such as skeletal, smooth, and cardiac muscles, and gain insights into their unique characteristics and roles within our body.

A. Muscle Contraction

Muscle contraction is the key process that allows muscles to generate force and produce movement. It is controlled by a complex interaction between nerve signals, calcium ions, and the proteins actin and myosin within the muscle fibers. When a nerve impulse reaches a muscle, it triggers the release of calcium ions, which bind to specific sites on the actin filament, leading to the sliding of actin and myosin filaments. This sliding action shortens the muscle fiber, resulting in contraction.

B. Motor Units

Motor units are the basic functional units of muscles. They consist of a motor neuron and the muscle fibers it innervates. When a motor neuron is stimulated, all the muscle fibers within its motor unit contract simultaneously. The size and number of motor units recruited to determine the force generated by a muscle. Fine movements require fewer and smaller motor units, while powerful movements involve the activation of more and larger motor units.

C. Energy Production

Muscle contractions require energy, which is supplied through the breakdown of adenosine triphosphate (ATP). The body utilizes different energy systems, such as the phosphagen system, glycolytic system, and oxidative system, to produce ATP during various types of physical activities. Each energy system has its characteristics and capacity to provide ATP, depending on the intensity and duration of the activity.

Understanding the intricate anatomy and physiology of muscles provides a foundation for comprehending their capabilities and limitations. It enables us to make informed decisions regarding training, nutrition, and overall muscle health. By delving into the complexities of muscle structure and function, we can optimize our training approaches and unlock the potential for enhanced performance and physical mastery.

Types of Muscle Fibers and Their Functions

Muscle fibers play a crucial role in determining our physical capabilities and performance. Within our skeletal muscles, there exist various types of muscle fibers, each with distinct characteristics and functions. This segment delves into the different types of muscle fibers, such as Type I, Type IIa, and Type IIb, exploring their specific attributes, endurance capacities, and force-generation abilities. Understanding these fiber types equips us with the knowledge needed to tailor our training and optimize muscle development.

Muscles are complex structures within our bodies that enable movement, provide stability, and support various bodily functions. Understanding the anatomy and physiology of muscles is fundamental to comprehending how they function and how we can optimize their performance.

A. Composition of Muscles

Muscles are made up of specialized cells called muscle fibers. These fibers are bundled together and surrounded by connective tissue, forming a muscle. The connective tissue extends beyond the muscle to form tendons, which attach muscles to bones. This arrangement allows muscles to transmit force and generate movement.

B. Organization of Muscles

Muscles are categorized into three main types: skeletal, smooth, and cardiac muscles. Skeletal muscles, also known as striated muscles, are attached to bones and control voluntary movements. Smooth muscles are found in the walls of organs and blood vessels, contributing to involuntary movements. Cardiac muscles are specific to the heart, enabling its rhythmic contractions.

Within our skeletal muscles, there are different types of muscle fibers, each possessing unique characteristics and functions. These muscle fiber types play a crucial role in determining our physical capabilities, endurance, and overall performance. Understanding the distinctions between these fiber types is essential for tailoring training programs and optimizing muscle development. Let's explore the various types of muscle fibers and their functions:

I. Type I (Slow-Twitch) Muscle Fibers

Type I muscle fibers are often referred to as slow-twitch fibers due to their relatively slower contraction speed. These fibers are highly resistant to fatigue and are primarily involved in activities that require endurance, such as long-distance running or cycling. Type I muscle fibers are rich in mitochondria, which provide the necessary energy for sustained contractions over extended periods. They are also efficient in utilizing oxygen and rely predominantly on aerobic metabolism. Type I fibers are responsible for maintaining posture and stability, making them crucial for activities that demand endurance and stability.

II. Type IIa (Fast-Twitch Oxidative) Muscle Fibers

Type II muscle fibers, also known as fast-twitch oxidative fibers, possess intermediate characteristics between Type I and Type IIb fibers. They exhibit a faster contraction speed than Type I fibers and possess a moderate resistance to fatigue. Type IIa fibers rely on a combination of aerobic and anaerobic metabolism to produce energy, making them suitable for activities that require both endurance and bursts of high-intensity effort. These fibers are involved in activities such as middle-distance running, swimming, and sports that demand a balance of speed and endurance.

III. Type IIb (Fast-Twitch Glycolytic) Muscle Fibers

Type IIb muscle fibers, also called fast-twitch glycolytic fibers, contract rapidly and generate high levels of force. They have a relatively larger diameter than Type I and Type IIa fibers. Type IIb fibers rely predominantly on anaerobic metabolism, making them ideal for short bursts of intense activity. However, they fatigue quickly compared to Type I and Type IIa fibers. Type IIb fibers are essential for explosive movements like sprinting, weightlifting, and other activities that require quick and powerful muscle contractions.

It's important to note that individuals have varying proportions of these muscle fiber types, which are determined by genetic factors and training adaptations. While the proportion of muscle fiber types is largely predetermined, targeted training can influence their size and performance characteristics to some extent.

Understanding the types of muscle fibers and their functions enables us to tailor our training strategies to suit our specific goals. Whether we aim to improve endurance, increase strength, or enhance overall athletic performance, knowledge of muscle fiber types empowers us to design training programs that optimize our genetic potential and promote targeted muscle development.

Muscle Growth and Adaptation

Muscle growth is a dynamic process driven by our body's response to physical stimuli. Whether we are athletes striving for peak performance or individuals seeking to improve their physiques, comprehending the principles of muscle growth and adaptation is crucial. This section elucidates the mechanisms behind muscle hypertrophy, examining factors such as resistance training, nutrition, and hormonal regulation. We delve into concepts such as muscle protein synthesis, satellite cells, and the importance of adequate recovery, providing valuable insights into optimizing muscle growth and adaptation.

By understanding the intricacies of muscle anatomy, the diverse characteristics of muscle fibers, and the mechanisms behind muscle growth and adaptation, we lay the groundwork for mastering our muscles. Armed with this knowledge, we can embark on a journey of intentional training, optimize our physical potential, and unlock the extraordinary capabilities that lie within our bodies.

Muscle growth, also known as muscle hypertrophy, is a complex process through which our muscles increase in size and strength. It is the result of a series of physiological adaptations that occur in response to the demands placed upon our muscles during exercise or physical activity. Understanding the mechanisms behind muscle growth and adaptation is crucial for anyone seeking to optimize muscle development and overall physical performance.

1. Resistance Training

Resistance training, often involving weightlifting or exercises that challenge our muscles against external resistance, is a primary stimulus for muscle growth. When we subject our muscles to progressive overload, meaning gradually increasing the intensity, volume, or difficulty of our workouts, it triggers a series of responses within the muscle fibers.

During our off seasons of athletic, our coach used to run on the sand and also climb slopes several times to strengthen our thigh muscles. This kind of resistance training always gave a power boost during actual competitions during cross-country races and track events.

2. Muscle Fiber Recruitment

During resistance training, our body recruits and activates muscle fibers to meet the demands of the exercise. The different types of muscle fibers, such as Type I (slow-twitch) and Type II (fast-twitch) fibers, are recruited based on the intensity and duration of the exercise. High-intensity, explosive exercises typically recruit Type II fibers, while endurance activities engage Type I fibers. Through consistent training, we can enhance the recruitment and activation of muscle fibers, leading to improved muscle growth and performance.

3. Muscle Protein Synthesis

One of the key mechanisms driving muscle growth is muscle protein synthesis (MPS). Resistance training stimulates MPS, which involves the creation of new muscle proteins to repair and rebuild damaged muscle fibers. This process requires an adequate intake of dietary protein, as protein serves as the building blocks for muscle repair and growth.

4. Hypertrophy and Satellite Cells

Muscle hypertrophy occurs when the size of individual muscle fibers increases, resulting in overall muscle growth. Resistance training causes microtrauma or small tears in the muscle fibers. In response to this damage, satellite cells, which are specialized cells located around muscle fibers, are activated. These satellite cells fuse with existing muscle fibers, donating their nuclei, and thereby contributing to the repair and growth of muscle fibers.

5. Hormonal Regulation

Hormones play a vital role in muscle growth and adaptation. Testosterone, growth hormone, insulin-like growth factor 1 (IGF-1), and insulin are among the hormones that influence muscle growth. Resistance training can increase the release of anabolic hormones, which promote muscle protein synthesis and overall muscle growth.

6. Recovery and Rest

Proper recovery and rest are essential for muscle growth and adaptation. When we engage in intense exercise, we create small disruptions in muscle fibers. Adequate rest and recovery allow these muscle fibers to repair and rebuild, leading to muscle growth. Sleep, nutrition, and managing overall stress levels are important factors that contribute to effective recovery and optimal muscle growth.

By understanding and applying these principles of muscle growth and adaptation, individuals can design effective training programs, tailor their nutrition, and optimize their recovery strategies. Consistency, progressive overload, and a holistic approach to training and lifestyle factors are key to achieving sustained muscle growth and maximizing overall physical performance.

Chapter Summary

"Understanding Your Muscles and Muscle Growth"

This chapter explores the essential aspects of muscles, their anatomy, physiology, and growth. It emphasizes the importance of comprehending muscle structure and function for optimizing physical performance and fitness. The chapter discusses muscle contraction, motor units, and energy production, providing insights into the mechanisms behind muscle movement. Additionally, it covers different types of muscle fibers (Type I, Type IIa, and Type IIb) and their roles in determining physical capabilities and performance. The final part of the chapter delves into muscle growth and adaptation, highlighting the significance of resistance training, muscle protein synthesis, hormonal regulation, and adequate recovery for optimizing muscle development and overall physical performance. Armed with this knowledge, readers can design effective training programs and unleash their true strength potential."

Next Chapter

Ready to unlock your strength potential? Dive into "The Science of Strength Training" chapter. Discover the scientific principles behind muscle adaptations, progressive overload, and optimal techniques. Get ready to train smarter, achieve remarkable results, and conquer new frontiers in your strength journey. The next chapter awaits!

Chapter 2

The Science of Strength Training

In the pursuit of mastering your muscles, understanding the science of strength training is paramount. We will discuss the scientific principles that form the foundation of effective strength training, providing you with the knowledge to optimize your workouts, stimulate muscle growth, and achieve exceptional results. By grasping these principles, you will unlock the key to transforming your physique and reaching new levels of strength and performance.

Principles of Strength Training

To embark on a successful strength training journey, it is crucial to grasp the fundamental principles that govern this discipline. This section explores concepts such as specificity, overload, and adaptation, helping you understand how to tailor your training to target specific muscle groups and achieve desired outcomes. By comprehending the principles of strength training, you will be able to design effective workout programs that maximize your efforts and yield remarkable results.

To embark on a successful strength training journey, it is essential to understand and apply the fundamental principles that underpin this discipline. These principles serve as guiding pillars, allowing you to design effective workouts, target specific muscle groups, and achieve optimal results. Let's explore the key principles of strength training:

Specificity

The principle of specificity emphasizes that training adaptations are specific to the type of exercise and the muscles involved. To maximize strength gains, it is important to focus on exercises that directly target the muscles you aim to develop. Tailor the training to reflect your specific goals, whether it is increasing overall strength, improving muscle endurance, or enhancing athletic performance.

Overload

The principle of overload states that for muscles to grow and get stronger, they must be exposed to a level of stress greater than what they are accustomed to. This involves progressively increasing the intensity, volume, or difficulty of your workouts over time. By challenging your muscles beyond their current capacity, you stimulate adaptations that result in muscle growth and improved strength.

Adaptation

The principle of adaptation highlights the body's remarkable ability to adapt to the demands placed upon it. When subjected to the stress of strength training, your muscles undergo physiological changes to become more resistant to future stress. This leads to muscle growth, increased strength, and improved performance. Consistency in training and allowing for proper recovery is crucial for optimal adaptation.

Individuality

The principle of individuality recognizes that each person responds differently to training stimuli. Factors such as genetics, age, gender, and training history can influence the rate and magnitude of strength gains. Tailor your training program to suit your unique needs, abilities, and limitations. Pay attention to how your body responds and make adjustments accordingly.

Variation

The principle of variation suggests that introducing variety in your training helps prevent plateaus and stimulates continuous progress. By regularly changing exercises, training methods, intensity levels, and rep ranges, you challenge your muscles in new ways, promoting ongoing adaptation and growth. Variation also keeps workouts engaging and enjoyable, reducing the risk of burnout or boredom.

Recovery

The principle of recovery emphasizes the importance of allowing your body adequate time to rest, repair, and rebuild between training sessions. Strength gains occur during recovery when the body repairs muscle tissue and replenishes energy stores. Insufficient recovery can hinder progress and increase the risk of overtraining and injury. Prioritize sleep, nutrition, and active recovery techniques to support optimal recovery and maximize your gains.

By applying these principles of strength training, you can design workouts that target specific muscle groups, progressively overload your muscles, and stimulate adaptations that lead to muscle growth and increased strength. Understanding these principles allows you to optimize your training, make consistent progress, and achieve your desired outcomes. Remember, mastering your muscles requires a thoughtful and strategic approach based on these fundamental principles of strength training.

Effective Workout Techniques for Muscle Growth

Building muscle is a primary objective of strength training, and employing the right workout techniques is vital to stimulate muscle growth. This segment dives into various effective techniques, including compound exercises, isolation exercises, and different training modalities like high-intensity interval training (HIIT) and circuit training. You will learn how to structure your workouts to target different muscle groups, create muscle tension, and optimize muscle fiber recruitment for optimal growth and development.

When it comes to muscle growth, employing the right workout techniques is essential to stimulate muscle fibers, promote hypertrophy, and achieve optimal results. This section explores various effective techniques that can be incorporated into your training regimen to maximize muscle growth and development.

1. Compound Exercises

Compound exercises are multi-joint movements that engage multiple muscle groups simultaneously. Examples include squats, deadlifts, bench presses, and pull-ups. These exercises recruit a large number of muscle fibers, providing a significant stimulus for growth. Incorporating compound exercises into your workouts allows you to target multiple muscle groups, increase overall strength, and stimulate greater muscle hypertrophy.

2. Isolation Exercises

Isolation exercises are single-joint movements that specifically target and isolate individual muscle groups. Examples include bicep curls, triceps extensions, and leg extensions. While compound exercises form the foundation of a strength training program, isolation exercises allow you to directly target and focus on specific muscles. By incorporating isolation exercises, you can achieve better muscle symmetry, address muscular imbalances, and enhance overall muscle definition.

3. Training Modalities

In addition to specific exercises, incorporating different training modalities can further enhance muscle growth. High-intensity interval training (HIIT) involves alternating between intense bursts of exercise and short recovery periods. HIIT workouts challenge both aerobic and anaerobic systems, leading to improved cardiovascular fitness and increased calorie burn, which can support fat loss while preserving muscle mass.

Circuit training involves performing a series of exercises with minimal rest in between. It provides a combination of resistance and cardiovascular training, promoting muscle endurance and conditioning. Circuit training is effective for individuals seeking to improve overall muscular fitness and enhance calorie expenditure during their workouts.

4. Volume and Intensity

Volume and intensity are important variables in designing effective workouts for muscle growth. Volume refers to the total amount of work performed in a training session and can be manipulated by adjusting sets, reps, and exercises. Increasing volume stimulates muscle fibers and promotes hypertrophy.

Intensity refers to the level of effort and load applied during exercises. By progressively increasing the intensity over time, such as by adding weight or reducing rest periods, you challenge your muscles and promote adaptation.

5. Periodization

A periodization is a strategic approach to organizing and varying training variables over specific periods. It involves dividing your training program into distinct phases, each with different training focuses and intensities. Periodization allows for progressive overload, prevents plateaus, and optimizes muscle growth and performance.

Remember, individual differences and goals should guide your choice of workout techniques. Consulting with a fitness professional or strength coach can help tailor these techniques to your specific needs and ensure proper form and execution.

By incorporating compound exercises, isolation exercises, utilizing different training modalities, manipulating volume and intensity, and implementing periodization strategies, you can create effective workout routines that maximize muscle growth. Consistency, proper form, and progressive overload remain key factors for success. Embrace these techniques, challenge your limits, and watch your muscles transform as you master your strength training journey.

Progressive Overload and Its Role in Building Muscle

Progressive overload is a key principle in strength training that drives muscle growth and adaptation. This section delves into the concept of progressive overload, which involves gradually increasing the demands placed on your muscles over time. You will learn how to manipulate variables such as intensity, volume, and frequency to continually challenge your muscles and elicit ongoing growth and strength gains. Understanding progressive overload empowers you to avoid plateaus and consistently make progress on your strength training journey.

By delving into the science of strength training, understanding the principles that drive muscle growth, and implementing effective workout techniques, you will be equipped with the tools to master your muscles. Whether you are a beginner looking to build a foundation of strength or an experienced athlete striving for new personal records, this information will provide you with the knowledge and strategies to optimize your strength training endeavors. Get ready to transform your physique, push your limits, and unlock your true strength potential.

Progressive overload is a fundamental principle in strength training and plays a vital role in building muscle. It refers to the gradual and systematic increase in the demands placed on your muscles over time. By consistently challenging your muscles with progressively higher levels of intensity, volume, or frequency, you stimulate muscle growth and adaptation. Here's a closer look at progressive overload and its significance in building muscle:

1. Stimulating Muscle Growth

Progressive overload is the key stimulus that prompts your muscles to grow stronger and larger. When you subject your muscles to a stressor that exceeds their current capacity, they respond by adapting to meet the increased demand. This adaptation occurs through various mechanisms such as increased protein synthesis, hypertrophy (muscle fiber enlargement), and enhanced neuromuscular coordination.

2. Increasing Training Intensity

One way to apply progressive overload is by gradually increasing the intensity of your workouts. This can be achieved by lifting heavier weights, performing more challenging variations of exercises, or increasing resistance through tools like resistance bands or weight plates. By consistently challenging your muscles with greater loads, you create micro-tears in the muscle fibers, triggering the repair and growth process.

3. Manipulating Training Volume

Training volume refers to the total amount of work performed during a workout, including sets, repetitions, and weight. Increasing training volume is another method of progressive overload. You can gradually add more sets or repetitions to your exercises or increase the overall workload within a given timeframe. This sustained increase in volume encourages greater muscle fiber recruitment, metabolic stress, and ultimately, muscle growth.

4. Adjusting Training Frequency

Training frequency refers to the number of times you train a specific muscle group or perform a particular exercise within a given time frame. Manipulating training frequency is another way to apply progressive overload. By gradually increasing the frequency of training sessions or dedicating more sessions to a specific muscle group, you provide additional stimuli for muscle growth and adaptation.

5. Tracking Progress

To effectively implement progressive overload, it's essential to track and monitor your progress over time. Keep a record of your workouts, including weights used, sets, reps, and any other relevant data. Regularly reassess your performance and make gradual adjustments to continue challenging your muscles. This ensures that you consistently apply progressive overload and avoid stagnation or plateaus.

Progressive overload is a dynamic and personalized process that needs to be tailored to your individual abilities, goals, and recovery capacity. It requires a progressive and systematic approach, allowing your muscles to adapt gradually to the increasing demands placed upon them. By implementing progressive overload intelligently and progressively, you can maximize muscle growth, strength gains, and overall performance in your strength training journey.

Chapter Summary:

"The Science of Strength Training"

This chapter explores the science behind strength training and its principles for optimal results. It emphasizes the importance of specificity, overload, adaptation, individuality, variation, and recovery.

Principles of Strength Training: Understanding the principles of strength training helps in designing effective workout programs. These principles include specificity, overload, adaptation, individuality, variation, and recovery.

Effective Workout Techniques for Muscle Growth: This section discusses various techniques for muscle growth, such as compound and isolation exercises, training modalities like HIIT and circuit training, and the importance of volume and intensity in designing workouts.

Progressive Overload and Its Role in Building Muscle: Progressive overload is a key principle in strength training. This section explains how gradually increasing the demands placed on muscles over time stimulates muscle growth and strength gains.

By mastering the science of strength training, employing effective workout techniques, and implementing progressive overload, individuals can optimize their strength training journey, stimulate muscle growth, and achieve their desired results.

Next Chapter

Take control of your fitness journey and design a personalized training program. Learn how to target specific muscle groups, optimize muscle growth, and enhance performance. Create a roadmap to success and unlock your true strength potential. Transform your physique and become the best version of yourself. Don't wait any longer, start designing your workout program now.

Chapter 3

Designing Your Workout Program

To make the most out of your fitness journey, it is crucial to have a well-designed workout program that aligns with your goals and suits your individual needs. Our discussion will guide you through the process of creating an effective workout plan that will help you master your muscles and achieve the results you desire. From setting goals and assessing your current fitness level to selecting the appropriate exercises for each muscle group, you will gain valuable insights and practical knowledge to design a personalized workout program that maximizes your potential.

Setting goals and assessing your current fitness level

Before diving into any workout routine, it is essential to set clear goals that will serve as your guiding light throughout your fitness journey. Whether your objective is to build muscle, lose weight, increase strength, or improve overall fitness, defining your goals will help you stay motivated and focused.

Assessing your current fitness level is another critical step in designing your workout program. It allows you to establish a baseline and determine where you stand in terms of strength, endurance, flexibility, and cardiovascular fitness. This self-assessment will help you identify your strengths and weaknesses, enabling you to tailor your program to address specific areas of improvement.

Remember, your first chapter can never be compared to the twenty-first of somebody else. Your schedule has to be fixed as per your standards. While undergoing competition at the state level and above I always followed the principles of my athletic coach who said if you are not placed in the competition, you must perform better than your previous best. We have to tear out during the competition but it is most important to watch your standard.

During the goal-setting and assessment process, consider factors such as time availability, commitment level, and any physical limitations or medical conditions you may have. Realistic and achievable goals combined with an honest assessment of your current fitness level will lay the foundation for an effective and sustainable workout program.

There is a certain exception when certain dedicated sports personalities set their standards high and work to the schedule. For instance, Usain Bolt has an extra bone growth in his right leg, which could have hindered his athletic career. Additionally, Bolt faced scoliosis, a condition that caused a slight curvature in his spine and left him with a leg half an inch shorter. Despite these obstacles, Bolt became the fastest man on earth, proving that determination and hard work can surpass any challenge.

Creating a personalized workout plan

Once you have established your goals and assessed your current fitness level, the next step is to create a personalized workout plan. A well-structured plan will ensure that you are targeting all the major muscle groups in your body while addressing your specific goals and needs.

When designing your workout plan, consider factors such as frequency (how often you will exercise), intensity (how hard you will work), duration (how long each session will last), and progression (how you will gradually increase the challenge over time). These variables can be adjusted based on your fitness level, preferences, and available time.

Additionally, it is important to incorporate a balance of cardiovascular exercise, resistance training, and flexibility work into your program. Cardiovascular exercise improves heart health and burns calories, while resistance training builds strength and muscle mass. Flexibility work enhances joint mobility and reduces the risk of injuries. By including all three components, you will achieve a well-rounded workout plan that promotes overall fitness and vitality.

Choosing the right exercises for different muscle groups

To effectively target different muscle groups, it is essential to select the appropriate exercises that activate and engage the specific muscles you want to work on. Understanding the anatomy and function of each muscle group will help you make informed choices when designing your workout routine.

There are various exercises available for each muscle group, ranging from compound movements that work multiple muscles simultaneously to isolation exercises that target specific muscles. Compound exercises, such as squats, deadlifts, and push-ups, are great for overall strength and functional fitness. Isolation exercises, such as bicep curls or triceps extensions, allow you to focus on a particular muscle group for more targeted growth and definition.

It is also important to vary your exercises to prevent boredom, challenge your muscles in different ways, and avoid overuse injuries. By incorporating a combination of free weights, machines, bodyweight exercises, and resistance bands into your routine, you can keep your workouts interesting and continuously challenge your muscles.

Remember, selecting the right exercises for different muscle groups should be based on your goals, fitness level, and equipment availability. By carefully choosing exercises that target specific muscles and incorporating variety into your routine, you will optimize muscle development and overall fitness.

Some of the specific weight training exercises may be suitable for weight lifters but they may not be generalized and practiced if you are a bodybuilder or athlete. Your workout and weight exercises should be chosen carefully as per the recommendations of experts.

By following the steps, you may gain the knowledge and skills necessary to design a workout program that is tailored to your goals, preferences, and abilities. A well-designed program will not only help you build strength and endurance but also ensure that you stay motivated and make consistent progress on your fitness journey.

Remember,

1. "A well-designed workout program is like a roadmap that leads you to your fitness goals."

2. "The key to success in fitness lies in designing a program that aligns with your goals and suits your individual needs."

Chapter Summary

"Designing Your Workout Program"

This chapter emphasizes the importance of creating a well-designed workout program tailored to your goals and needs. It covers setting goals, assessing your current fitness level, and creating a personalized plan. The plan should include factors like frequency, intensity, duration, and progression. It should also incorporate a balance of cardiovascular exercise, resistance training, and flexibility work. Choosing the right exercises for different muscle groups is crucial, considering factors such as muscle activation and variety. By following these steps, you can design a program that promotes strength, endurance, and consistent progress on your fitness journey.

Next Chapter

This chapter provided valuable insights on designing an effective workout program tailored to your goals and needs. Now, it's time to move on to the next chapter: "Fueling Your Muscles." In this chapter, you will discover the importance of nutrition and proper fueling for optimal performance and muscle development. Let's explore the secrets to maximizing your workout results by delving into the world of fueling your muscles for success!

Chapter 4

Fueling Your Muscles

To achieve optimal muscle development, it is crucial to understand the role of nutrition in fueling your muscles. Nutrition plays a vital role in providing the necessary building blocks for muscle growth, repair, and recovery. Without proper nutrition, even the most rigorous workouts may fail to yield the desired results. Let us discuss the importance of nutrition for muscle development and provide insights into the macronutrients that are essential for fueling muscle growth. Furthermore, we will explore pre-and post-workout nutrition strategies that can enhance your muscle-building efforts and help you achieve your fitness goals.

The role of nutrition in muscle development

Nutrition forms the foundation for muscle development. When it comes to building and maintaining muscle mass, exercise alone is not sufficient. Adequate nutrition provides the essential nutrients, vitamins, and minerals that support muscle growth and repair. It is through the consumption of specific nutrients that your body can synthesize new muscle tissue, repair damaged muscle fibers, and optimize overall muscle function. You will learn in detail the highlights or the significance of proper nutrition in facilitating muscle development and discuss the key nutrients that contribute to this process.

You may be vegetarian or non-vegetarian; you can choose your diet accordingly. Here are some examples of foods that are natural sources of protein, which can be beneficial for gym goers:

1. Lean meats

Chicken breast, turkey breast, lean beef, and pork tenderloin are excellent sources of high-quality protein.

2. Fish

Salmon, tuna, trout, and other fatty fish provide not only protein but also omega-3 fatty acids, which have numerous health benefits.

3. Eggs

Whole eggs, including the egg yolk, are a complete source of protein and contain essential amino acids.

4. Dairy products

Greek yogurt, cottage cheese, and whey protein are rich in protein, making them suitable options for gym enthusiasts.

5. Legumes

Lentils, chickpeas, black beans, and other legumes are plant-based protein sources that are also high in fiber.

6. Quinoa

This pseudo-grain is a complete protein source and contains all nine essential amino acids. It's a great alternative to rice or pasta.

7. Tofu and tempeh

Both tofu and tempeh are soy-based products and are popular among vegetarians and vegans due to their high protein content.

8. Nuts and seeds

Almonds, walnuts, chia seeds, and flaxseeds are examples of protein-rich foods that also provide healthy fats and other beneficial nutrients.

9. Quorn

Quorn is a meat substitute made from mycoprotein, a type of fungus. It's a low-fat, high-protein option often used by vegetarians and vegans.

10. Protein-rich vegetables

Broccoli, spinach, Brussels sprouts, and peas are examples of vegetables that contain a notable amount of protein.

Remember that the protein requirements can vary depending on individual needs, so it's important to consult a nutritionist or dietitian to determine the appropriate intake for your specific goals and circumstances.

Macronutrients and their importance for muscle growth

I used to take whey protein during the day to compensate the muscle recovery. However, I was taking it at different periods. On the suggestion of my expert trainer, I started taking it within the first 10 to 15 minutes as post workout diet and it proved to be the best for muscle gain.

Macronutrients, namely proteins, carbohydrates, and fats, are the primary sources of energy for your body. Each macronutrient plays a distinct role in muscle growth and maintenance. Proteins, for example, are the building blocks of muscle tissue and are essential for muscle repair and growth. Carbohydrates provide energy for intense workouts and replenish muscle glycogen stores. Fats play a crucial role in hormone production and aid in nutrient absorption. Let us delve into the specific roles of proteins, carbohydrates, and fats in muscle growth and provide guidelines for incorporating them into your diet for optimal results.

Pre-and post-workout nutrition strategies

At least three hours of a gap was suggested by the trainer to undergo workouts and it was advised to have some fruits like apples or bananas before the workout.

The timing and composition of your meals surrounding your workouts can significantly impact your muscle-building progress. Pre- and post-workout nutrition strategies aim to maximize muscle protein synthesis, minimize muscle breakdown, and optimize recovery. It is very much essential to know the importance of pre-workout nutrition in providing the energy and nutrients necessary for an effective workout. It will also explore post-workout nutrition, emphasizing the importance of consuming the right combination of macronutrients to replenish energy stores, initiate muscle repair, and promote muscle growth. Additionally, we will provide practical tips and guidelines for implementing effective pre-and post-workout nutrition strategies to enhance your muscle-building efforts.

By understanding the critical role of nutrition in muscle development and adopting appropriate strategies for fueling your muscles, you can optimize your training results and unlock your full potential. Let's dive into the world of muscle fueling and empower ourselves to master our muscles.

Remember,

1. "Your muscles are like an engine, and proper nutrition is the fuel that powers them to reach their full potential."

2. "To build strong muscles, you need to give them the right fuel - the right nutrients at the right time."

Chapter Summary

"Fueling Your Muscles"

Fueling Your Muscles focuses on the role of nutrition in muscle development and offers strategies for optimizing your diet to support muscle growth and recovery. It emphasizes that exercise alone is insufficient and highlights the importance of proper nutrition in providing the building blocks for muscle growth, repair, and function. The significance of macronutrients, such as proteins, carbohydrates, and fats, is explained, along with guidelines for incorporating them into your diet. Pre- and post-workout nutrition strategies are explored to maximize muscle protein synthesis and promote muscle repair and growth. By understanding and implementing these strategies, you can optimize your muscle-building efforts and achieve your fitness goals.

The Next Chapter

Are you eager to discover the secrets of maximizing muscle recovery? If so, don't miss out on the next chapter, "Maximizing Muscle Recovery." This chapter delves into effective techniques and strategies to optimize your body's ability to recover and rebuild after intense workouts. Discover the importance of rest, proper nutrition, and targeted recovery methods that can accelerate your muscle repair and growth. Uncover the key principles that will help you bounce back stronger, reduce the risk of injury, and achieve peak performance. Don't miss the chance to unlock the secrets of maximizing muscle recovery. Turn the page and embark on the next step of your fitness journey!

Chapter 5

Maximize Muscle Recovery

"The magic happens outside your comfort zone, but the recovery happens inside it."

- Roland Carlstedt

There is a critical role of rest and recovery in promoting muscle growth. We have to know certain techniques that can optimize the recovery between workouts, ensuring that we bounce back stronger and achieve our fitness goals. There is a profound impact of sleep and stress management on muscle development. Let us uncover the secrets of maximizing muscle recovery and take the training to the next level.

1. The importance of rest and recovery for muscle growth

Rest and recovery are fundamental aspects of muscle development. When you engage in intense workouts, you create microscopic tears in your muscle fibers. It is during the recovery phase that these fibers repair and grow stronger. Adequate rest allows your body to replenish energy stores, reduce inflammation, and optimize the synthesis of new muscle proteins.

Austrian-American actor, bodybuilder Arnold Schwarzenegger once said,

"Strength and growth come only through continuous effort and struggle. But the key to success lies in the ability to recover and adapt."

Let us understand the importance of rest through these examples.

A. Rest days

Incorporate dedicated rest days into your training routine, allowing your muscles time to recover and rebuild. This could involve light activities like stretching, yoga, or simply taking a day off from structured workouts.

B. Active recovery

Engage in low-impact activities such as swimming, cycling, or leisurely walks, which promote blood flow and aid in muscle recovery without causing excessive stress.

2. Techniques to optimize recovery between workouts

To maximize muscle recovery, it's important to implement various techniques that enhance the body's ability to repair and rebuild. These techniques aim to reduce muscle soreness, inflammation, and fatigue, allowing you to bounce back quickly for your next training session.

You can employ some of the techniques as follows.

A. Foam rolling

Use a foam roller to perform a self-myofascial release, targeting tight or sore muscles. This helps alleviate muscle tension and promotes better blood circulation.

B. Stretching

Incorporate static and dynamic stretches into your post-workout routine to improve flexibility and reduce muscle stiffness.

C. Contrast water therapy

Alternate between hot and cold-water immersion, such as a hot shower followed by a cold shower or an ice bath. This technique can aid in reducing inflammation and promoting muscle recovery.

3. Sleep, stress management, and their impact on muscle development

Sleep and stress management plays crucial roles in muscle development. Quality sleep allows the body to repair and regenerate, while chronic stress can hinder muscle growth and recovery.

One of my junior managers in my previous organization spent almost 2 to 3 hours in the gym regularly, diet was also observed with the quality required however, he had a minor heart attack. The age was 38 years. It was found from the observation of the medical team that he was taking sleep only for 5 hours for the last four months.

It has been proved by experts that sleep inertia can have various effects on cognitive function, including reduced attention, decreased memory performance, and impaired decision-making. It can also affect physical coordination and increase the risk of accidents or errors immediately after awakening.

Let us understand the vital importance of an adequate amount of sleep and prioritize sleep.

Aim for 7-9 hours of uninterrupted sleep each night. Create a conducive sleep environment, establish a regular sleep routine, and practice relaxation techniques like deep breathing or meditation before bed. Some of the experts also mention reading a few pages of self-help books before sleeping. The exclusive ideas of eminent authors' experiences fill the mind with positivity, cultivation of a growth mindset, and success in life.

4. Stress management

Incorporate stress-reducing activities into your daily routine, such as practicing mindfulness, engaging in hobbies, or spending time in nature. These activities help lower cortisol levels, which can impede muscle growth.

By recognizing the significance of rest, implementing recovery techniques, prioritizing sleep, and managing stress effectively, you can optimize your muscle recovery. Remember, allowing your body to heal and rebuild is just as important as the intensity of your workouts. Stay tuned for the next chapter as we continue to explore the art of mastering your muscles.

Here are three stress management techniques we can implement in daily life.

A. Deep Breathing

Deep breathing is a simple and effective technique to quickly reduce stress. Take slow, deep breaths, inhaling through your nose and exhaling through your mouth. Focus on filling your abdomen with air as you breathe in, and then slowly release the breath. Deep breathing helps activate the body's relaxation response, calming your mind and reducing stress levels.

B. Exercise

Engaging in physical activity is an excellent way to manage stress. Regular exercise releases endorphins, which are natural mood-boosting chemicals in the brain. It can help reduce anxiety, improve your mood, and increase your overall sense of well-being. Find an activity you enjoy, whether it's going for a walk, jogging, dancing, or practicing yoga, and aim for at least 30 minutes of exercise most days of the week.

C. Mindfulness or Meditation

Mindfulness and meditation practices can help you cultivate a greater sense of calm and clarity. By focusing your attention on the present moment, you can reduce stress and enhance your ability to cope with challenges. You can start by finding a quiet space, sitting comfortably, and bringing your attention to your breath or a specific object. Allow your thoughts and emotions to come and go without judgment, bringing your focus back whenever your mind starts to wander.

It's important to find what works best for you and to make stress management a regular part of your routine. If your stress levels persist or become overwhelming, it may be helpful to seek support from a healthcare professional or therapist.

Points To Ponder

1. "The true power of a workout lies in the recovery. Treat your body well, nourish it, and allow it to repair and grow stronger."

2. "Recovery is not a sign of weakness; it's an essential part of the process. Embrace rest and let your muscles rebuild and replenish."

3. "Recovery is where progress is made. Take the time to rest, recharge, and allow your muscles to rebuild. It's the secret to long-term gains."

Chapter Summary

"Maximizing Muscle Recovery,"

This chapter highlights the vital role of rest and recovery in muscle growth. It emphasizes the repair and strengthening of muscle fibers during the recovery phase. The importance of incorporating rest days and engaging in active recovery activities is discussed. Techniques such as foam rolling, stretching, and contrast water therapy are introduced to optimize recovery. The impact of sleep and stress management on muscle development is emphasized, encouraging readers to prioritize sleep and incorporate stress-reducing activities. By understanding the significance of rest, implementing recovery techniques, and managing sleep and stress, readers can enhance their muscle recovery for better results.

Next Chapter

The next chapter will deal with innovative methods to elevate your fitness regimen. Discover cutting-edge strategies to enhance strength, endurance, and overall performance. From supersets and drop sets to pyramid training and eccentric training, this chapter explores advanced techniques that push your boundaries and stimulate new muscle growth. Unleash the power of progressive overload, leverage tempo variations, and embrace advanced training protocols. Prepare to take your workouts to the next level as you unlock the secrets of advanced training techniques. Turn the page and embark on an exciting journey of physical transformation.

Chapter 6

Advanced Training Techniques

Let us explore the realm of some advanced training techniques, designed to challenge your muscles and take your fitness journey to new heights. These techniques go beyond traditional workouts and provide innovative ways to maximize your gains. By incorporating high-intensity interval training (HIIT), supersets, drop sets, and other intensity techniques, as well as integrating plyometrics and functional movements, you will unleash the full potential of your muscles and achieve remarkable results.

1. High-intensity interval training (HIIT)

HIIT is a time-efficient and highly effective training method that alternates between short bursts of intense exercise and brief recovery periods. By pushing your limits during intense intervals, you elevate your heart rate, increase calorie burn, and boost your metabolism. HIIT not only improves cardiovascular fitness but also enhances muscle strength and endurance. Incorporating exercises like sprints, jump squats, and burpees, HIIT stimulates muscle growth and promotes overall athleticism.

Let us understand with a couple of examples.

A. Tabata Training

Tabata training is a popular form of HIIT that follows a specific interval structure. It consists of 20 seconds of intense exercise followed by 10 seconds of rest, repeated for a total of 8 rounds (4 minutes). You can choose any exercise that gets your heart rate up, such as burpees, mountain climbers, or squat jumps. Perform the exercise at maximum effort during the 20-second intervals and rest during the 10-second intervals. This intense burst of exercise followed by short recovery periods boosts cardiovascular fitness and improves muscular endurance.

B. Sprint Intervals

Sprint intervals involve alternating between periods of all-out sprinting and active recovery. Find a track, treadmill, or outdoor space where you can sprint safely. Start with a warm-up, then sprint at maximum effort for a predetermined distance, such as 100 meters, and follow it with a recovery period of walking or slow jogging. Repeat this cycle for a desired number of rounds or times, gradually increasing the intensity and duration as your fitness improves. Sprint intervals enhance cardiovascular capacity, burn calories, and promote muscular strength and power.

During the workout in the evening, our athletic coach of the defence organization used to give 10 rounds of running on 400 meters track with a couple of minutes rest. These repetitions induced a high level of cardio training required for representing long-distance events and cross-country competitions.

It's important to modify the exercises and intensity based on your fitness level and consult with a healthcare professional before starting any new exercise program.

2. Supersets, drop sets, and other intensity techniques

Supersets and drop sets are advanced intensity techniques that challenge your muscles by combining different exercises or adjusting the weight and repetitions within a set. Supersets involve performing two exercises back-to-back without rest, targeting different muscle groups or the same muscle group from different angles. Drop sets, on the other hand, involve gradually reducing the weight while maintaining the same exercise, pushing your muscles to fatigue. These techniques increase the intensity, maximize time under tension, and promote muscle hypertrophy and strength gains.

Here are some intensity techniques for supersets, drop sets, and other intensity techniques:

A. Pre-Exhaust Supersets

Instead of pairing two different exercises, pre-exhaust supersets involve performing a compound exercise followed immediately by an isolation exercise targeting the same muscle group. For example, start with a set of barbell squats (compound exercise) and immediately follow it with a set of leg extensions (isolation exercise) to specifically target your quadriceps. This technique fatigues the target muscle group with the compound exercise and then isolates it further with the subsequent exercise, maximizing muscle recruitment and promoting muscle growth.

B. Mechanical Drop Sets

Mechanical drop sets involve changing the resistance or the exercise variation within a set to continue working for the muscle group after fatigue sets in. Start with a challenging weight or exercise variation, and as you reach muscle failure, immediately switch to a lighter weight or an easier variation to allow for continued repetitions. For example, during a bicep curl, you could start with a dumbbell and then switch to a resistance band once you reach fatigue. This technique prolongs the intensity of the set and pushes your muscles to their limits.

C. Rest-Pause Sets

Rest-pause sets involve taking short rest periods within a set to extend the total number of repetitions and increase time under tension. Choose a weight that challenges you and perform as many repetitions as possible. When you reach fatigue and can no longer complete full repetitions, pause for a few seconds (10-15 seconds) to catch your breath and regain some strength. Then, continue with more repetitions until you reach fatigue again. Repeat this process for a desired number of rest-pause cycles. Rest-pause sets enhance muscle endurance and stimulate muscle growth.

3. Drop Set Descending Pyramid

In a drop set descending pyramid, you start with a heavy weight and gradually decrease the weight as you continue the set. Begin with a weight that allows you to perform 6-8 reps with proper form. After reaching muscle failure, immediately reduce the weight by around 20-30% and continue the set with another 6-8 reps. Repeat this process, decreasing the weight and performing another set of reps until you can no longer complete the desired range. This technique provides continuous stimulation to the muscles and induces metabolic stress, contributing to muscle growth and development.

Remember, when incorporating these intensity techniques, ensure proper form, use appropriate weights, and listen to your body's signals. Gradually increase the intensity and weight as your strength improves, and always prioritize safety and proper technique during your workouts.

4. Incorporating plyometrics and functional movements

Incorporating plyometrics and functional movements into your training involves engaging in dynamic exercises that enhance power, agility, and overall functional fitness. Plyometrics focus on explosive movements that rapidly stretch and contract muscles, such as box jumps, jump lunges, or medicine ball throws. These exercises improve muscular power, speed, and coordination while targeting multiple muscle groups simultaneously. Functional movements, on the other hand, are inspired by everyday activities and aim to improve strength, stability, and mobility. Exercises like squats, deadlifts, and lunges mimic real-life movements, enhancing overall functional fitness and helping you perform daily tasks with greater ease. By incorporating plyometrics and functional movements, you can develop athleticism, improve muscular coordination, and enhance your overall physical performance.

Plyometrics, also known as jump training, involves explosive movements that rapidly stretch and contract muscles, such as box jumps, jump lunges, or medicine ball throws. These dynamic exercises enhance power, speed, and agility while engaging multiple muscle groups simultaneously. Functional movements, inspired by everyday activities, focus on improving strength, stability, and mobility through exercises like squats, deadlifts, and lunges. By incorporating plyometrics and functional movements into your training, you improve athletic performance, develop muscular coordination, and enhance overall functional fitness.

By exploring and implementing these advanced training techniques, you will break through plateaus, challenge your body in new ways, and stimulate continuous muscle growth and development. Remember to prioritize proper form, listen to your body, and gradually progress as you embrace the power of advanced training methods.

Prepare to master your muscles and unlock your full potential with these cutting-edge techniques.

Chapter Summary

"Advanced Training Techniques,"

In this chapter, we explored innovative methods to challenge your muscles and optimize your fitness journey. We begin by incorporating high-intensity interval training (HIIT), which alternates between intense exercise and brief recovery periods to boost cardiovascular fitness, increase calorie burn, and improve muscle strength and endurance. Examples such as Tabata training and sprint intervals illustrate how to implement HIIT effectively.

Next, we delve into intensity techniques like supersets, drop sets, and others. Supersets involve performing exercises back-to-back without rest, targeting different muscle groups or angles. Drop sets gradually reduce weight to prolong the set and push muscles to fatigue, promoting muscle hypertrophy and strength gains. Techniques such as pre-exhaust supersets, mechanical drop sets, and rest-pause sets are introduced to maximize intensity and stimulate muscle growth.

Lastly, we explore incorporating plyometrics and functional movements. Plyometrics involves explosive movements like box jumps and jump lunges to enhance power, speed, and coordination. Functional movements, inspired by everyday activities, improve strength, stability, and mobility through exercises like squats and deadlifts.

By embracing these advanced training techniques, you will overcome plateaus, stimulate muscle growth, and unlock your full potential. It is crucial to prioritize proper form, listen to your body, and gradually progress. Get ready to master your muscles and achieve remarkable results through these cutting-edge techniques.

Next Chapter

We will now proceed to the next chapter and learn strategies to break through stagnant periods and conquer obstacles that may hinder your progress. Discover effective techniques to overcome plateaus, adapt your training, and push beyond your limits. From adjusting your workout routine and implementing progressive overload to exploring new training modalities and seeking professional guidance, this chapter provides insights and solutions to help you navigate and conquer challenges on your fitness journey. Turn the page and embark on a transformative chapter that will propel you toward continued growth and success.

Chapter 7

Overcoming Plateaus and Challenges

In the pursuit of building and sculpting our muscles, we often encounter hurdles that impede our progress and leave us feeling frustrated and stagnant. Plateaus, injuries, and setbacks are common challenges faced by fitness enthusiasts on their muscle-building journey. However, with the right understanding and strategies, we can overcome these obstacles and continue progressing toward our goals. We will now explore the common muscle-building plateaus, discuss effective strategies to break through stagnation, and critically evaluate and deal with injuries and setbacks during the fitness journey.

Understanding common muscle-building plateaus

Plateaus are periods where our muscle growth seems to come to a halt, and despite our best efforts, we struggle to make further progress. Let us understand the various types of plateaus commonly encountered in muscle-building.

Strength Plateau

A strength plateau refers to a phase in your muscle-building journey where you experience a significant slowdown or complete halt in your ability to increase the amount of weight you can lift or the number of repetitions you can perform. It is a frustrating phase characterized by a lack of progress in terms of raw strength gains.

During the initial stages of strength training, you may notice rapid improvements as your muscles adapt and grow stronger. However, as you continue to push your limits and approach the peak of your natural strength potential, you are more likely to encounter a strength plateau.

Several factors can contribute to a strength plateau, including:

1. Neural Adaptation:

Initially, your strength gains are primarily due to improvements in neural adaptations, such as increased recruitment of motor units and improved coordination. However, once your neural system becomes more efficient, further progress in strength becomes more challenging.

2. Muscle Adaptation:

Over time, your muscles adapt to the stress placed upon them, becoming more resistant to further growth. This adaptation occurs as your muscles become better at handling the specific demands of your training routine.

3. Insufficient Progressive Overload:

Progressive overload, which involves gradually increasing the demands placed on your muscles, is vital for continued strength gains. If you fail to consistently challenge your muscles with progressively heavier weights or higher training volumes, you may reach a plateau.

Overcoming a strength plateau requires implementing effective strategies to stimulate further strength gains. Some strategies to consider include:

1. Adjusting Training Variables:

Manipulating training variables such as intensity, volume, and rest periods can help break through a strength plateau. Incorporating techniques like drop sets, supersets, and pyramid sets can provide a new stimulus to your muscles.

2. Periodization:

Implementing a well-structured periodization plan can help you systematically vary the intensity and volume of your workouts. This approach allows for planned periods of higher and lower-intensity training, facilitating continued progress and preventing plateaus.

3. Incorporating Different Exercises:

Introducing new exercises or variations of existing exercises can target your muscles from different angles and recruit different muscle fibers, challenging your body in new ways and stimulating further strength gains.

4. Prioritizing Recovery:

Sufficient rest and recovery are crucial for overcoming a strength plateau. Ensure you are getting adequate sleep, fueling your body with proper nutrition, and allowing for regular rest days to allow your muscles to repair and grow stronger.

Remember, breaking through a strength plateau requires patience, consistency, and a willingness to challenge yourself. By implementing these strategies and remaining dedicated to your training regimen, you can overcome the strength plateau and continue progressing toward your strength goals.

Size Plateau

Here, our muscle growth seems to plateau, and we struggle to add more size or mass to our muscles despite consistent training and proper nutrition.

A size plateau refers to a phase in your muscle-building journey where you struggle to add more size or mass to your muscles, despite consistent training and proper nutrition. It is a frustrating period characterized by a lack of visible muscle growth or an inability to increase muscle size.

Various factors can contribute to a size plateau:

1. Genetic Factors:

Genetics play a significant role in determining muscle size potential. Some individuals may naturally have a greater capacity for muscle growth, while others may find it more challenging to build significant muscle mass.

2. Adaption to Training Stimulus:

Over time, your muscles adapt to the specific demands of your training routine. Initially, you may experience rapid muscle growth as your body responds to the new stimulus. However, as your muscles become more accustomed to the exercises and training volume, further growth becomes more difficult.

3. Inadequate Progressive Overload:

Progressive overload, which involves progressively increasing the intensity or volume of your workouts, is crucial for stimulating muscle growth. If you fail to challenge your muscles with progressively heavier weights, additional repetitions, or increased training volume, your muscles may reach a plateau.

To overcome a size plateau and continue building muscle mass, consider implementing the following strategies:

1. Progressive Overload:

Ensure that you are consistently increasing the demands placed on your muscles. Gradually increase the weights you lift, add more repetitions, or incorporate advanced training techniques like drop sets or rest-pause sets. This progressive overload will provide a new stimulus for muscle growth.

2. Variation in Training:

Introduce variety into your training routine to shock your muscles and prevent them from adapting to the same stimulus. This can include changing exercise selection, altering training methods (e.g., using free weights instead of machines), or incorporating different training modalities like resistance bands or bodyweight exercises.

3. Focus on Compound Exercises:

Compound exercises, such as squats, deadlifts, bench presses, and rows, involve multiple muscle groups and stimulate overall muscle growth. Prioritize these compound movements in your workouts to target a larger number of muscle fibers and promote muscle size gains.

4. Ensure Proper Nutrition:

Muscle growth requires adequate nutrition, particularly a sufficient intake of protein to support muscle repair and growth. Ensure you are consuming enough protein-rich foods and maintaining an overall caloric surplus to support muscle growth.

5. Sufficient Recovery:

Allow your muscles enough time to rest and recover between workouts. This allows for muscle repair and growth. Aim for quality sleep, manage stress levels, and consider incorporating active recovery strategies such as stretching or foam rolling.

By implementing these strategies and remaining consistent and patient, you can break through a size plateau and continue progressing toward your muscle-building goals. Remember that each individual's journey is unique, and results may vary. Focus on long-term progress and maintaining a sustainable approach to training and nutrition.

Endurance Plateau

Endurance plateaus can be frustrating when we find ourselves unable to improve our muscular endurance, making it challenging to sustain intense workouts or perform high-repetition exercises.

An endurance plateau refers to a phase in your muscle-building journey where you struggle to improve your muscular endurance. It is a period characterized by an inability to sustain intense workouts or perform high-repetition exercises without experiencing fatigue or a decrease in performance.

Several factors can contribute to an endurance plateau:

1. Lack of Training Variety:

If your workouts consistently focus on low-repetition, high-intensity exercises, your muscles may become accustomed to this specific type of training. As a result, they may not adapt to the demands of higher-repetition exercises or sustained bouts of endurance-based training.

2. Inadequate Training Volume:

Insufficient training volume can hinder improvements in muscular endurance. If your workouts do not include enough sets, repetitions, or time under tension, your muscles may not be adequately challenged to improve their endurance capacity.

3. Limited Cardiovascular Fitness:

Muscular endurance is not solely dependent on your muscles; it also relies on your cardiovascular system's ability to deliver oxygen and nutrients to the working muscles. If your cardiovascular fitness is lacking, it can hinder your endurance progress.

To overcome an endurance plateau and enhance your muscular endurance, consider implementing the following strategies:

1. Increase Training Volume:

Gradually increase the number of sets, repetitions, or time under tension in your workouts. This progressive increase in training volume challenges your muscles to adapt and improve their endurance capacity.

2. Incorporate High-Rep Training:

Include exercises or workouts that specifically target higher repetitions. Focus on exercises that engage multiple muscle groups, such as circuit training or high-intensity interval training (HIIT), which can improve both cardiovascular fitness and muscular endurance.

3. Implement Supersets or Drop Sets:

Incorporate supersets, where you perform two exercises back-to-back without rest, or drop sets, where you gradually reduce the weight as you reach fatigue, into your workouts. These techniques can help increase training intensity and challenge your muscles to work at higher levels of endurance.

4. Engage in Cardiovascular Training:

Include regular cardiovascular exercises such as running, cycling, swimming, or rowing to improve your overall cardiovascular fitness. Enhancing your cardiovascular capacity can positively impact your muscular endurance.

5. Rest and Recovery:

Adequate rest and recovery are essential for allowing your muscles to repair and adapt. Ensure you have appropriate rest days between intense workouts to prevent overtraining and optimize your endurance progress.

6. Proper Nutrition and Hydration:

Maintain a balanced diet that includes sufficient carbohydrates for energy and protein for muscle repair. Proper hydration is also crucial for optimal endurance performance.

By implementing these strategies and maintaining consistency in your training, you can overcome an endurance plateau and improve your muscular endurance. Remember that progress takes time, so be patient and stay focused on your long-term goals.

Understanding these different plateaus is crucial as it allows us to tailor our strategies to specifically target the underlying causes and overcome the stagnation.

Strategies to break through stagnation and keep progressing

When faced with plateaus, it is important to implement effective strategies that can reignite our progress and push past these obstacles. we will now explore various strategies that can help us break through stagnation:

a) Progressive Overload:

Understanding the concept of progressive overload and how to implement it is crucial for continuous muscle growth. We will discuss techniques such as increasing weight, adding repetitions, and manipulating training variables to challenge our muscles and stimulate further growth.

b) Variation in Training:

Introducing variety into our training routine can prevent plateaus by shocking our muscles with new stimuli. We will explore techniques such as changing exercise selection, altering training volume and intensity, and incorporating different training modalities.

c) De-loading and Recovery:

Proper recovery is essential for muscle growth. We can consider the importance of incorporating de-load periods and adequate rest to prevent overtraining and breakthrough plateaus.

Dealing with injuries and setbacks during your fitness journey

Injurics and setbacks are unfortunate but common occurrences in any fitness journey. It is crucial to approach them with the right mindset and strategies to ensure a speedy recovery and minimal disruption to our progress. Let us explore to know subject injuries in detail.

a) Injury Prevention:

Exploring techniques and practices that can help minimize the risk of injuries during training, such as proper warm-up routines, correct form and technique, and listening to our bodies.

b) Rehabilitation and Recovery:

When injuries do occur, it is important to focus on effective rehabilitation techniques, including proper rest, targeted exercises, and seeking professional guidance, if necessary, to ensure a safe and efficient recovery.

c) Mental Resilience:

Dealing with setbacks requires mental strength and resilience. We will discuss strategies to stay motivated, maintain a positive mindset, and adapt our training approach during challenging times.

By understanding these strategies and approaches, we can navigate through the plateaus, injuries, and setbacks that may arise during our muscle-building journey, ensuring continued progress and achieving our desired results.

Chapter Summary

"Overcoming Plateaus and Challenges"

In this chapter, we explored the common muscle-building plateaus, discuss strategies to break through stagnation and address injuries and setbacks in the fitness journey.

Understanding common muscle-building plateaus:

We also discussed different types of plateaus encountered in muscle-building, including strength plateaus, size plateaus, and endurance plateaus. We explore the factors contributing to each plateau and gain a deeper understanding of the challenges faced.

Strategies to break through stagnation and keep progressing:

To overcome plateaus, we discussed effective strategies such as progressive overload, variation in training, and adequate recovery. These techniques help challenge muscles, introduce new stimuli, and prevent stagnation.

Dealing with injuries and setbacks during your fitness journey:

We addressed the unfortunate occurrences of injuries and setbacks and provided insights on injury prevention, rehabilitation, and recovery. Mental resilience strategies are also discussed to navigate challenging times.

By implementing these strategies and understanding the causes of plateaus and setbacks, we can overcome obstacles, continue progressing, and achieve our muscle-building goals.

The Next Chapter

Let us now read the next chapter "The Role of Mindset in Muscle Transformation" and explore how developing a positive and empowered mindset can significantly impact your muscle-building journey.

Chapter 8

The Role of Mindset in Muscle Transformation

In the pursuit of physical transformation, the role of mindset cannot be overstated. While exercise routines, nutrition plans, and rest are crucial elements in the journey to sculpting our bodies, the power of the mind is often overlooked. The way we think and perceive ourselves, our goals, and our abilities can significantly impact the results we achieve. Let us discuss the effects of the profound influence of mindset on muscle transformation, exploring how a positive mental approach can enhance our progress and help us overcome obstacles.

1. Harnessing the power of a positive mindset

A positive mindset is a potent tool that can unlock our true potential. When we believe in ourselves and our capacity for growth, we can push beyond perceived limitations and reach new heights. By adopting a positive mindset, we cultivate self-belief, resilience, and the determination to overcome challenges.

For example, imagine an individual who begins their muscle transformation journey with a negative mindset, constantly doubting their ability to succeed. They may start skipping workouts, making excuses, and giving in to self-defeating thoughts. On the other hand, someone with a positive mindset approaches their training with enthusiasm, determination, and a belief that they can achieve their goals. This individual consistently shows up to their workouts, pushes through tough moments, and stays committed to their nutrition plan. The power of a positive mindset lies in its ability to fuel consistent action and sustain long-term progress.

One thing I have found in my psychological studies is that if someone keeps an avoidance goal in mind, there is an ill effect of the exercise and workout. For instance, one can speak as follows,

"If I go to the gym, I may not get diabetes or high blood pressure."

This is the wrong kind of affirmation. Instead, one can speak as follows,

"If I train myself regularly in the gym, I can be very happy and healthy." We can avoid undesirable words in affirmation or conversation. You can avoid words like stress, tragedy, depression, and more in daily conversation as far as it is possible.

2. Visualizations, affirmations, and mental conditioning

Visualizations, affirmations, and mental conditioning techniques are valuable tools that harness the power of the mind to facilitate muscle transformation. By vividly picturing the desired outcome and reinforcing positive beliefs, we can align our subconscious mind with our conscious goals.

For instance, visualizations involve mentally imagining ourselves with the muscular physique we aspire to achieve. By regularly visualizing our desired results during workouts or through meditation, we create a powerful connection between our mind and body. This mental rehearsal helps improve focus, motivation, and overall performance.

Affirmations play a vital role in shaping our mindset. By repeating positive statements about our capabilities and progress, we reinforce empowering beliefs. For example, repeating affirmations such as "I am strong, I am capable, and dedicated to transforming my body" can bolster self-confidence and provide a mental boost during challenging workouts or moments of self-doubt.

Mental conditioning techniques, such as creating pre-workout rituals or using specific cues, can help establish a positive mindset before training sessions. These techniques signal to the brain that it's time to shift into a focused, determined state. This preparation primes the mind for optimal performance, enabling individuals to fully engage in their workouts and make the most of their efforts. Our subconscious mind understands two languages. One is the command language and another is images. If you continuously focus and see certain images daily, it makes a deep impression on your mind. It will become real. In the same way, when things are repeated in speech, things happen. If we speak positively, positive things will happen, and if negative things are repeated, negative things happen. The subconscious mind does not distinguish between negative and positive. It treats the things same. So, we should always speak positively.

3. Overcoming self-doubt and staying motivated

Self-doubt is a common obstacle that can hinder progress in muscle transformation. It can undermine our confidence, make us question our abilities, and lead to inconsistency or even giving up altogether. Overcoming self-doubt requires a strong mindset and effective strategies for staying motivated.

One powerful approach is to challenge and reframe negative self-talk. For example, instead of thinking, "I can't lift that heavy weight," we can shift our mindset to "I am working toward increasing my strength, and with consistent effort, I will get there." By reframing negative thoughts and focusing on the process of growth, we can gradually silence self-doubt and foster a more positive and empowering inner dialogue.

Additionally, setting realistic goals and celebrating milestones along the way can help maintain motivation. Breaking down the larger transformation goal into smaller, achievable targets provides a sense of progress and accomplishment. Recognizing and celebrating these milestones serves as positive reinforcement, further fueling motivation and perseverance.

In conclusion, the power of mindset in muscle transformation cannot be underestimated. A positive mindset, fueled by visualizations, affirmations, and mental conditioning techniques, helps us overcome self-doubt and stay motivated. By harnessing the power of our thoughts and beliefs, we unlock our true potential, enabling us to achieve remarkable physical transformations.

Remember some,

1. "The most significant muscle you can train in the gym is your mind. A positive mindset empowers you to conquer any obstacle and transform your body into its greatest form."
2. "Challenges are an inevitable part of muscle transformation, but a resilient mindset turns obstacles into stepping stones towards success."

Chapter Summary

"The Role of Mindset in Muscle Transformation,"

We learned the importance of mindset in achieving successful physical transformations. While exercise routines, nutrition, and rest play crucial roles in sculpting the body, the power of the mind is often overlooked. A positive mindset acts as a potent tool, enabling individuals to push beyond perceived limitations and achieve their goals.

Also, we discussed the effects of a positive mindset on muscle transformation, exploring various ways it can enhance progress and overcome obstacles. It highlights the significance of visualizations, affirmations, and mental conditioning techniques in aligning the subconscious mind with conscious fitness goals. By vividly picturing the desired outcome, reinforcing positive beliefs, and establishing pre-workout rituals, individuals can improve focus, motivation, and overall performance.

Later on, we addressed the challenge of self-doubt, which can hinder progress. To overcome self-doubt, the chapter suggests reframing negative self-talk and focusing on the process of growth. Setting realistic goals and celebrating milestones along the way can further maintain motivation and perseverance.

We then emphasized that a positive mindset is essential in achieving remarkable physical transformations. By harnessing the power of thoughts and beliefs, individuals can unlock their true potential and conquer any obstacle on their journey to a stronger, healthier body.

Next Chapter

Now, let's embark on an equally exciting and vital phase of your fitness journey

"Sustaining Your Muscular Transformation Strategies."

In this next chapter, you will discover essential techniques to maintain and build upon the progress you've made so far. Learn how to make fitness a sustainable lifestyle, ensuring lasting results and continued growth. From effective workout regimens to smart nutrition choices, these strategies will empower you to keep your hard-earned gains and take your muscle transformation to new heights. So, don't miss out on the opportunity to solidify your success and dive into the secrets of sustaining a fit, healthy, and transformed physique! Let's get started on the next chapter right away!

Chapter 9

Sustaining Your Muscular Transformation

If you have come a long way in your fitness journey, now it may be the time to focus on the next phase: maintaining your hard-earned gains for the long term. Sustaining your progress requires dedication, determination, and a strategic approach. We will now, explore essential strategies to keep you on track, ensuring your muscles remain strong, toned, and ready for any challenge that comes your way. Remember, this is not just about looking good; it's about embracing a lifestyle that empowers you to thrive in every aspect of your life. Let's dive in and discover the power of perseverance and the art of muscular maintenance.

Incorporating Variety and Periodization in Your Training

Variety is the spice of life, and it's no different in the world of fitness. To sustain your muscular transformation, you must constantly challenge your muscles with different stimuli. Mixing up your workouts not only keeps things exciting but also prevents your body from plateauing. Periodization is a powerful tool that will take your training to new heights.

Incorporate different training modalities like strength training, hypertrophy-focused workouts, plyometrics, and functional movements. Embrace the challenge of trying new exercises and training methods. Engage in resistance training with varying rep ranges, intensity, and rest periods.

Periodization involves structuring your training program into distinct phases, each with its unique focus and intensity. This approach optimizes muscle adaptation and recovery while minimizing the risk of overtraining. From high-volume training to strength-focused blocks, periodization allows you to continually progress and evolve.

Meet Sarah, a fitness enthusiast who has just completed her muscular transformation journey. She recognizes that maintaining her progress requires a fresh approach to her workouts. Sarah decides to mix things up by incorporating different training modalities. She includes strength training for building muscle mass, plyometric exercises for explosive power, and functional movements to enhance her overall athleticism. Additionally, Sarah embraces periodization and structures her training program into distinct phases. She spends a few weeks focused on hypertrophy, followed by a strength-focused block to challenge her muscles in new ways. The result? Sarah's progress remains steady, and she never falls into the trap of monotony.

Balancing Muscle Development with Overall Health and Well-being

While striving for muscle gains, it's crucial not to lose sight of your overall health and well-being. Sustainability comes from finding harmony between fitness and self-care. Your muscular transformation journey should empower you, not consume you.

Incorporate rest days into your weekly routine to allow your muscles to recover and grow. Remember, rest is not a sign of weakness but a vital aspect of progress. Restorative practices like yoga and meditation can enhance your mind-muscle connection, reduce stress, and promote better sleep.

Nutrition is the foundation of your muscular maintenance. Fuel your body with wholesome, nutrient-dense foods that nourish your muscles and support your energy levels. Stay hydrated to optimize your performance and overall health.

Meet Mike, a dedicated fitness enthusiast who has seen tremendous muscle gains over the past year. However, Mike recognizes that his progress is not just about lifting weights but also about taking care of his body and mind. To ensure he sustains his muscular transformation, Mike incorporates rest days into his weekly routine. On these days, he engages in gentle yoga and meditation to enhance his recovery and reduce stress levels. Moreover, Mike pays close attention to his nutrition, making sure to fuel his body with nutrient-dense foods. He prioritizes sleep, staying hydrated, and focuses on overall well-being. This balanced approach allows Mike to maintain his muscle gains while feeling energized and empowered in all aspects of his life.

Emotional and Mental Strength for Long-Term Success

Muscle maintenance goes beyond the physical; it requires emotional and mental fortitude. Your mindset plays a significant role in sustaining your transformation. Cultivate a positive attitude and embrace the journey, with all its ups and downs.

Set realistic and achievable goals, both short-term and long-term, and celebrate every milestone along the way.

Surround yourself with a supportive community or training partner who can motivate and inspire you when the going gets tough.

Visualize your success, see yourself maintaining your muscular transformation, and let that vision fuel your determination. You've already proven to yourself that you can achieve greatness, so keep that fire alive and push through any obstacles that may come your way.

Example: Let's meet Alex, who has gone through an incredible muscular transformation journey. However, like any fitness journey, Alex faces challenges and setbacks. To sustain his progress, he understands that his mental strength is just as crucial as his physical prowess. Alex cultivates a positive attitude and refuses to be deterred by obstacles. Whenever he encounters a tough day in the gym or faces a temporary plateau, he reminds himself of how far he's come and visualizes his long-term success. Alex also seeks support from his training partner, who motivates and encourages him to keep pushing forward. With unwavering determination and a powerful mindset, Alex conquers any hurdles that come his way, ensuring his muscular transformation is not just a momentary achievement but a lifelong commitment to excellence.

Conclusion

Sustaining your muscular transformation is a testament to your strength, both physically and mentally. By incorporating variety and periodization into your training, you keep your body primed for continuous growth. Remember always to prioritize overall health and well-being, making rest and nutrition an integral part of your routine.

With emotional resilience and a positive mindset, you'll conquer any challenges that come your way, and your muscular transformation will become a lifelong journey of growth and self-discovery. Embrace the power of perseverance, and let your muscles be a reflection of the strength that resides within you.

Chapter Summary

"Sustaining Your Muscular Transformation"

In this chapter, we emphasized the importance of maintaining your hard-earned gains for the long term. To ensure success, dedication, determination, and a strategic approach are essential. The chapter explores strategies to keep your muscles strong, toned, and ready for any challenge. Variety is key in sustaining your transformation. Constantly challenge your muscles with different stimuli to prevent plateaus. Embrace different training modalities like strength training, plyometrics, and functional movements. Implement periodization to structure your program into distinct phases, optimizing muscle adaptation and recovery. Harmony between fitness and self-care is crucial. Incorporate rest days, restorative practices like yoga, and nutrient-dense foods into your routine. Prioritize hydration and sleep for optimal performance and overall health. Mental fortitude is vital for sustaining progress. Cultivate a positive attitude, set realistic goals, and celebrate milestones. Visualize your success, seek support from a community or partner, and push through obstacles with unwavering determination. Maintaining your muscular transformation is a testament to both physical and mental strength. With variety, periodization, and a balanced approach to health, you'll thrive in your fitness journey. Embrace the power of perseverance and let your muscles reflect the strength within you, leading to a lifelong commitment to excellence and self-discovery.

Last Chapter

As you continue your journey towards sustaining your muscular transformation and maximizing your fitness potential, I encourage you to explore the valuable insights and wisdom found in the last chapter, "The Exemplary Traits of an Extraordinary Trainer." This chapter delves into the qualities that set apart exceptional trainers and coaches, those who can truly elevate your fitness experience and empower you to achieve greatness. From their motivational prowess to their ability to tailor training programs to individual needs, these extraordinary trainers will undoubtedly inspire you to new heights in your fitness journey. So, let's dive into the world of exceptional coaching and unlock the secrets to unlocking your full potential. Head over to the final chapter now and unleash the greatness within you!

Chapter 10

The Exemplary Traits of an Extraordinary Trainer

Not everyone can become a trainer. It requires unwavering dedication, tenacious commitment, and unyielding motivation. I am thrilled to showcase the remarkable dedication and commitment of a few exceptional trainers from our fitness center in Ahmedabad. These trainers hold a special place in my heart, and their stories are truly inspiring.

Qualities of a good trainer

Here are some general good qualities of a good or expert trainer that can inspire you.

1. **Knowledgeable:** A good trainer possesses extensive knowledge and expertise in their field. They stay updated with the latest research, techniques, and trends in fitness and can provide accurate and reliable information to their clients.

2. **Excellent Communication Skills:** Effective communication is crucial for a trainer. They can explain complex concepts clearly and concisely,

3. ensuring that clients understand the instructions and guidelines properly. They also actively listen to their client's concerns, questions, and feedback.

4. **Adaptability:** A good trainer understands that each individual is unique and has different goals, abilities, and limitations. They can adapt their training methods and programs to suit the specific needs of their clients. They are flexible in their approach and can modify exercises, routines, and techniques as required.

5. **Motivational:** Motivation is a key factor in achieving fitness goals. A good trainer knows how to inspire and motivate their clients to push beyond their limits and stay committed to their fitness journey. They provide encouragement, support, and positive reinforcement, helping clients stay focused and determined.

6. **Personalized Approach:** A good trainer recognizes that a one-size-fits-all approach doesn't work for everyone. They take the time to assess each client's individual needs, goals, and abilities and design personalized training programs accordingly. They consider factors such as fitness level, medical history, preferences, and lifestyle to create tailored plans.

7. **Safety-Conscious:** Safety is a top priority for a good trainer. They prioritize proper form, technique, and safety precautions during workouts to minimize the risk of injuries. They educate their clients about correct exercise execution and ensure that clients are using appropriate equipment and weights.

8. **Passionate and Enthusiastic:** A good trainer is passionate about fitness and genuinely cares about their client's well-being. They radiate enthusiasm and energy, which helps motivate and inspire their clients. Their passion for what they do is infectious, creating a positive and engaging training environment.

9. **Professionalism:** A good trainer maintains a high level of professionalism in their interactions with clients. They are punctual, organized, and respectful of their client's time. They maintain confidentiality and adhere to ethical guidelines in their practice.

10. **Continuous Learner:** A good trainer is committed to their own professional development and continuous learning. They actively seek out opportunities to expand their knowledge, attend workshops, pursue certifications, and engage in

ongoing education to stay at the forefront of their field.

11. **Empathy and Emotional Intelligence:** A good trainer understands the emotional and psychological aspects of the fitness journey. They empathize with their clients' struggles, challenges, and setbacks. They possess emotional intelligence and are skilled at building rapport, understanding their clients' motivations, and providing the necessary support and encouragement.

While going through a remarkable journey to the gym for the last couple of years, I have met a few trainers who have possessed these qualities and changed my fitness to the next level. Let me introduce some of them to you.

Trainer: Prashant Mudliyar

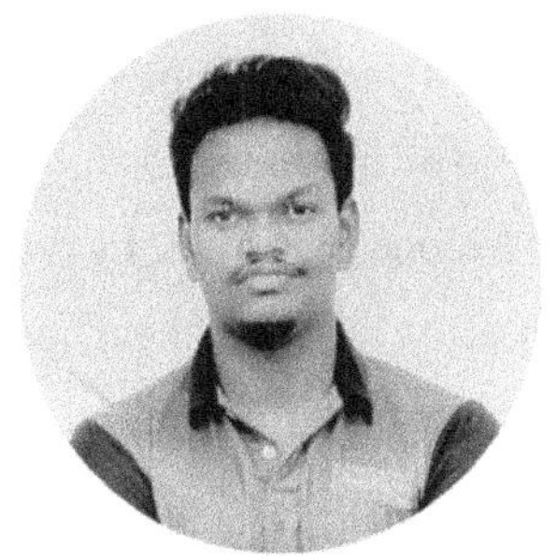

Meet Prashant Mudliyar, a trainer whose dedication to fitness is unparalleled. Despite recently experiencing a severe leg injury in an accident, Prashant continued to show up at the center, providing guidance and instructions to trainees, even on the most trivial matters. Despite his struggles to walk, he motivated everyone to stick to their fitness routines. His unyielding commitment led him to become a certified advanced personal trainer, specializing in various categories after studying at the renowned Gold Gym Fitness Institute. We witnessed countless trainees lose anywhere from 10 to 18 kilograms under his guidance. Prashant, a commerce graduate from a prestigious university, has been serving the fitness community for over six years. In addition to his expertise in fitness, he has acquired proficiency in five different languages, showcasing his exceptional communication skills.

Prashant's commitment level is unmatched and unparalleled. He firmly believes in pushing boundaries and inspiring his clients to surpass their limits. With meticulous precision, he designs personalized training programs tailored to each individual's goals and abilities. Prashant ensures that his clients not only achieve their desired results but also develop a deep and lasting passion for fitness that extends beyond the confines of the gym.

His infectious enthusiasm and positive energy serve as a constant source of inspiration to those around him. Prashant possesses a profound understanding of the mental and emotional challenges that accompany physical transformations, and he employs various motivational techniques to keep his clients engaged and driven. His clients often describe him as an unwavering motivator who consistently pushes them to strive for excellence.

Words cannot adequately express our gratitude for Prashant's selfless service and unwavering efforts. He exemplifies the true spirit of a dedicated trainer, and his impact on lives is immeasurable.

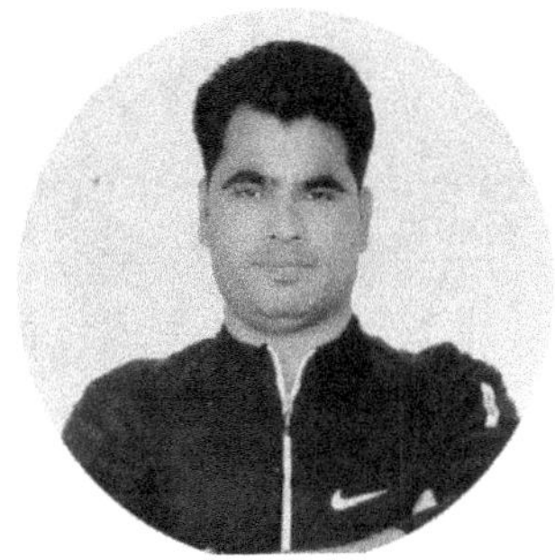

Trainer: Jignesh Borana

Jignesh Borana is a true proponent of the intricate mind-body connection. He firmly believes that physical strength and mental well-being are interdependent. With a background in scriptwriting and motivational videos, coupled with extensive training in various fitness disciplines, Jignesh brings a distinctive approach to his coaching. He holds a degree from a prestigious university and boasts an impressive 15 years of experience in the field.

Jignesh's commitment to his clients' holistic well-being is nothing short of remarkable. He places great emphasis on achieving balance, encouraging his clients to cultivate mindfulness, self-compassion, and self-awareness alongside their physical training. His sessions are carefully crafted to address not only the physical aspects but also mental resilience, stress management, and overall emotional health.

Under Jignesh's guidance, clients embark on transformative journeys that extend beyond mere physical changes. They report heightened self-confidence, improved focus, and a renewed sense of purpose in their lives. Jignesh's dedication to helping individuals harness the power of the mind-body connection truly sets him apart. Notably, his specialization in weight loss and bodybuilding has garnered him exceptional recognition.

Trainer: Shant Chauhan

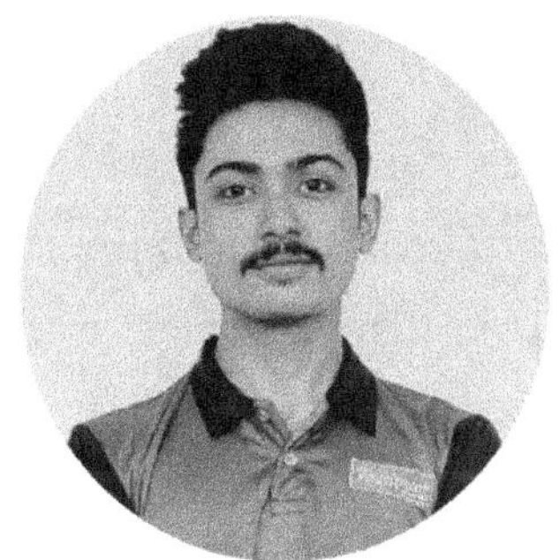

Shant Chauhan, the epitome of youthful vitality, brings his elite athletic training experience to his clients. His unwavering commitment to fitness stems from his formative years of rigorous training and competing at the highest echelons of athletic achievement. Renowned for his relentless work ethic and unwavering pursuit of excellence, Shant's dedication to pushing boundaries is unparalleled. Furthermore, Shant holds a bachelor's degree in Sports Management (BBA) and boasts four years of invaluable training experience.

Driven by a burning desire to help his clients achieve greatness, Shant sets exceptionally high standards for both himself and those he trains. He meticulously designs rigorous training programs that challenge the physical and mental limits of his clients. His unyielding commitment to their success serves as a constant source of motivation, compelling clients to surpass their expectations.

Shant's impact extends beyond physical training as he assumes the role of mentor, guiding clients through the peaks and valleys of their fitness journeys. Instilling in them the values of discipline, perseverance, and resilience that he acquired during his athletic career, Shant is credited by his clients for not only transforming their bodies but also shaping their character.

The combination of Shant's unwavering dedication, exceptional expertise, and mentorship distinguishes him as an exceptional trainer and an invaluable asset to his clients' fitness journeys.

Trainer: Jay Acharya

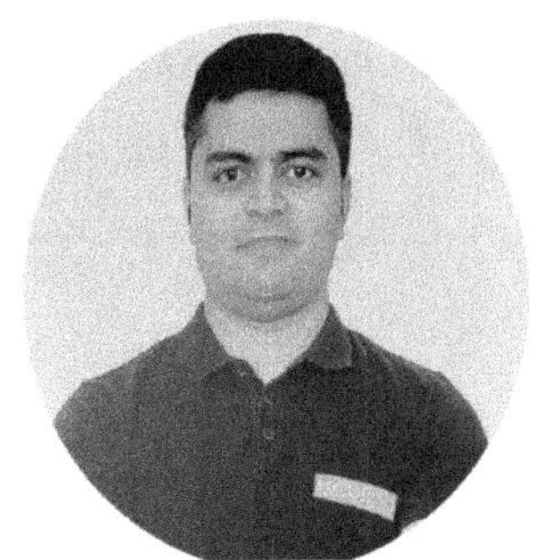

In the vibrant corridors of the fitness center, amidst the clatter of weights and lively conversations, a remarkable figure stood tall, embodying unwavering dedication and unyielding commitment. This is the tale of Jay Acharya, an extraordinary trainer who has profoundly transformed the lives of over 500 individuals, igniting greatness through 17 years of remarkable experience. As we embark on his journey, we delve into the depths of perseverance and the relentless pursuit of excellence. It is worth noting that Jay Acharya holds a master's degree (M.Sc.) in Bioinformatics.

His exceptional degree endows students with a unique fusion of biological knowledge, computational skills, and statistical expertise. This broad range of capabilities allows Jay to assume versatile roles within the fitness industry, enabling him to assist trainees with an extensive understanding of healthcare, genetics, and more. His expert knowledge consistently contributes to comprehending and solving complex biological queries using computational methods whenever required by clients.

Jay's story commences not amidst the spotlight, but within the quiet recesses of his self-discovery. From an early age, Jay was drawn to physical activities, finding solace and purpose within the confines of the gymnasium. The seed of passion was planted, and it blossomed into an insatiable fire that fueled his every stride.

A truly remarkable trainer is not solely defined by his physical prowess but by the breadth of his knowledge. Jay's thirst for comprehending the intricacies of the human body led him on an eternal quest for wisdom. Through countless hours of research, certifications, and workshops, he refined his expertise, establishing himself as an unparalleled authority in the field.

Within the bustling fitness center, Jay assumed the role of more than just a trainer; he became a guiding beacon, illuminating the path toward self-improvement for all who sought his guidance. His unwavering dedication to the well-being of his clients resonated in every session, propelling each individual beyond his perceived limits with empathy, encouragement, and an unwavering belief in his untapped potential.

The transformative power of consistent dedication should never be underestimated. Jay's influence extended far beyond the walls of the gymnasium, permeating the lives of his clients. Through his unwavering support, countless individuals discovered the strength to conquer their doubts, redefine their boundaries, and embark on a lifelong journey of self-discovery and personal growth.

Jay Acharya's story encapsulates the essence of dedication, commitment, and the indispensable role he plays in transforming lives. His unyielding determination and unwavering pursuit of excellence continue to inspire all who cross his path. Jay's tale serves as a poignant reminder that with dedication and commitment, one can truly master his physical capabilities and unlock the boundless potential within.

It is widely acknowledged, even among his fellow trainers, that Jay Acharya is a pioneer in weight loss, specialized population training, and scientifically grounded nutrition.

Due to various exceptional skills, he works as a branch manager of the fitness center.

I thank all the above trainers from the bottom of my heart.

Conclusion

Pain points of gym goers and tentative solutions

There are a lot of pain points for gym enthusiasts. A single book may not be sufficient for resolving the issues however with the help of a few trainers I found some issues and I give a single liner solution to such issues.

Lack of Motivation:

Solution: Find a workout buddy or hire a personal trainer to provide accountability and encouragement. Set achievable goals and reward yourself for reaching milestones.

Plateau in Progress:

Solution: Vary your workouts regularly to keep challenging your muscles. Incorporate new exercises, increase weights, or try different training techniques like supersets or drop sets.

Muscle Soreness and Recovery:

Solution: Prioritize rest and recovery days. Incorporate stretching, foam rolling, and light activities like walking or yoga to improve circulation and reduce soreness.

Ensure proper nutrition and hydration for optimal recovery.

Time Constraints:

Solution: opt for high-intensity interval training (HIIT) or circuit workouts that provide effective results in less time. Plan and schedule workouts in advance to make them a priority.

Lack of Knowledge and Guidance:

Solution: Take advantage of gym orientation sessions or hire a personal trainer to design a customized workout plan based on your goals and fitness level.

Monotony and Boredom:

Solution: Join group exercise classes or try different fitness activities like dance, martial arts, or sports to keep workouts exciting and enjoyable.

Fear of Injury:

Solution: Focus on proper form and technique during exercises. Start with lower weights and gradually increase as your strength and confidence grow. Seek guidance from fitness professionals to ensure safe and effective workouts.

Gym Intimidation:

Solution: Remind yourself that everyone starts somewhere and most people are focused on their workouts. Gradually become familiar with the gym layout and equipment. Consider off-peak hours to avoid crowds.

Lack of Results:

Solution: Track your progress with measurements, photos, or fitness apps to see improvements over time. Adjust your workout and nutrition plan if necessary or seek professional guidance to address potential obstacles.

Cost of Gym Memberships:

Solution: Explore more affordable options, such as community centers or outdoor fitness classes. Create a home workout space with basic equipment or bodyweight exercises.

Balancing Work and Exercise:

Solution: Incorporate small bouts of physical activity throughout the day, like taking short walks during breaks or using a standing desk. Find ways to combine exercise with other tasks, such as biking to work.

Body Image Concerns:

Solution: Focus on overall health and well-being rather than just appearance. Set realistic and achievable fitness goals and celebrate non-scale victories.

Lack of Progress Tracking:

Solution: Keep a workout journal or use fitness apps to track your workouts, nutrition, and progress. Seeing your improvements can boost motivation and provide insights for further adjustments.

However, individual pain points can vary, and these solutions are general suggestions. It's essential to listen to your body and seek personalized advice from fitness professionals when needed.

I wish my readers a very healthy life ahead.

Bibliography

- Million Dollar Habits, Brian Tracy

- Goals, Brian Tracy

- Awaken Giant Within, Tony Robbins

- My life, Dr. APJ Kalam

Acknowledgment

I am very much thankful to branch manager admin of the fitness point for providing me various useful information.

About the Author

The author boasts 15 years of commendable service in the Indian Air Force in technical stream, specializing in Aero Engines for a range of aircraft utilized by the Armed Forces. He excelled in the role of an Engine Fitter, with a particular expertise in Helicopter engines. Throughout his tenure, he was stationed in diverse locations across the country, including the challenging terrains of Leh-Ladakh and Jammu and Kashmir. His contributions to the Armed Forces encompassed pivotal operations such as Blue Star Operation, Blast Track Operation, and Passive Air Defense during peacetime. Not limited to the Air Force, he also lent his expertise to the Army, serving in Air Defence Regiments. In addition to his knowledge of aircraft and equipment, he received training in the handling of firearms such as .303 rifles and LMGs. While involved in aircraft maintenance, he assumed the responsibilities of a Guard Commander, ensuring the utmost security levels at various Air Force units. As a senior noncommissioned officer, he supervised the operations of canteen store departments and unit run canteens. He published his military biography, "What I Will Be Remembered For," which not only portrays his personal journey but also sheds light on the remarkable accounts of wartime operations and introduces readers to the realm of gallantry awards.

Following his tenure in the Indian Air Force, the author pursued a successful 24-year career in the supervisory cadre of the State Bank of India, where he held positions such as Field Officer, Account Officer, and Branch Manager in several branches across Gujarat state Of India. Demonstrating exemplary performance, he effectively managed and upgraded multiple branches to the status of being recognized as "Exceptionally Well Run," meeting the bank's high standards. During his diverse assignments, he skillfully supervised teams and resources, motivating his subordinates to achieve optimal results. As a Joint Custodian of the Reserve Bank of India, he ensured the smooth flow of cash for ATM replenishments and the Currency Administrative Cells of both SBI branches and other banks. In recognition of his outstanding managerial skills, he was awarded the title of Best Branch Manager of the State Bank of India for the year 2014-15.

Moreover, the author holds a master's degree in Psychology, which he earned in 1986 from a prestigious university in South India. Throughout his active service in the Armed Forces and corporate sector, he guided organizations and individuals, drawing upon his extensive experiments and experiences, to effectively resolve day-to-day challenges. To enhance his skill set, he pursued courses in computer studies, obtaining diplomas in DISM and PGDCA from Saurashtra University, as well as completing a program at APTECH. Alongside his banking career, he dedicated his spare time to teaching students, conducting morning and evening classes where he imparted knowledge on MS Office, C++, Visual FoxPro, Visual Basics, and website designing.

Beyond his professional accomplishments, the author indulges in various artistic pursuits, including vocal and instrumental performances on the harmonium, guitar, flute, mouth organ, and violin. Having showcased his talents on All India Radio, he has graced stages across different regions of Gujarat. Presently, the author is actively engaged in producing a diverse range of content, including books and videos on topics spanning banking, meditation, motivation, music, and exploring the profound effects of personality traits and attitudes on human behavior, thereby delving into the fascinating realm of human psychology.

*****